Wilson Reading System®

Student Reader
One

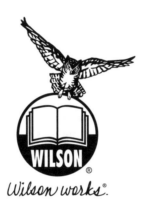

THIRD EDITION

by Barbara A. Wilson

Wilson Language Training Corporation

www.wilsonlanguage.com

Wilson Reading System® Student Reader One

Item # SR1AB

ISBN 978-1-56778-067-3

THIRD EDITION (revised 2004)

PUBLISHED BY:

Wilson Language Training Corporation
47 Old Webster Road
Oxford, MA 01540
United States of America

(800) 899-8454

www.wilsonlanguage.com

Printed in the U.S.A.

November 2011

Step 1 Concepts

Closed Syllables (3 sounds)

1.1   **f, l, m, n, r, s** (initial) · **d, g, p, t** (final) · **a, i, o** (blending of 2 and 3 sounds)

1.2   **b, sh** · **u** · **h, j** · **c, k, ck** · **e** · **v, w, x, y, z** · **ch, th** · **qu, wh** (introduced gradually)

1.3   Practice with above sounds (**wish, chop, wet**)

1.4   Double consonants, **all** (**bill, kiss, call**)

1.5   **am, an** (**ham, fan**)

1.6   Adding suffix **-s** to closed syllable words with 3 sounds (**bugs, chills**) *a* | *s, m, r* (initial) | *d, g, p, t* (final)

sad	sat	sap
mad	mat	map
rat	rag	rap

rap	map	sat
sap	sad	mad
mat	rat	rag

The rat is mad.

The rat sat on the mat.

The rat had a rag.

f, l, m, n, r, s (initial) | *d, g, p, t* (final)

lap	lad	lag
nap	nag	Nat
fat	map	rat

Matt	rag	rap
lap	sad	mat
nap	fat	sat

Nat is sad.

Is the fat rat on his lap?

The rag is on the mat.

a | *f, l, m, n, r, s* (initial) | *d, g, p, t* (final)

rap	Nat	rag
sat	sap	mat
lag	nag	sad

Matt	lap	map
lad	fat	at
nap	rat	mad

Matt had a nap.

Nat is sad.

The lad had the map.

i

rip	rid	rig
lip	lit	lid
sip	sit	Sid

fit	lid	lit
rip	it	rid
sit	Sid	sip

The rag had a rip.

Did Sid sit on the map?

The lid fit.

i, a

fit	fig	fat
sit	sip	sat
lip	lid	lap

fit	it	Nat
map	sip	lid
rag	nip	lap

Matt had a sip.

Is Nat mad at Sid?

Sid had a nap on the mat.

a, i, o

rod	rot	rat
not	nod	nap
lot	log	lap

fog	not	lot
on	log	Rod
rot	rod	mop

It is not a rat.

Rod sat on the log.

Matt had the mop.

a, i, o

fog	lot	rap
nod	not	nag
mop	lot	fit

Rod	rip	rap
rot	rat	mat
rag	sag	log

Did the log rot?

The map is on his lap.

Sid is not in the lot.

b (final) | *sh*

Rob	mob	nab
sob	rib	fib
lab	rob	lob

fish	lash	rash
shot	shop	mash
ship	shag	Nash

Rob had a rash.

The ship had a lot of fish on it.

Matt Nash had to shop.

u

lug	mug	rut
mutt	rush	sun
run	mud	sub

mud	mug	map
sun	sub	sat
rush	run	rash

Sid is in a rush.

Rob sat in the sun.

Matt had a sip from the mug.

b, d, g, p, t (initial)

pig	pit	pat
tap	tag	top
dog	dot	dig

bag	bat	bit
gap	gash	got
big	dug	bug

The dog had a dish of fish.

The bug is in the pot.

Pat had a pig in the pit.

b, d, g, p, t (initial)

gum	pot	pad
dash	tug	bud
tot	tip	dish

Pat	pup	bus
dug	but	dad
bad	bun	pop

Did Bud run to the shop?

The pup sat in the sun.

The tot got gum on the rug.

a, i, o, u | *b, d, f, g, l, m, n, p, r, s, t, sh*

1 Sal got a lot of fish.

2 The bus is in a rut.

3 Did the dog dig the pit?

4 Dash to the shop for a sub.

5 The gum is in the bag.

6 Dad had a bad rash.

7 The bat is in his lap.

8 Rob bit the fig but did not like it.

9 Mom had a sip of pop.

10 Did Tim mop the shop?

h, j

hop	hit	hush
hat	hot	hip
hid	hog	had

job	jug	jot
jut	jab	Jim
jig	jog	jag

Jim got the job on the ship.

Did Mom jog to the shop?

The tot hid the hat.

c, k

cat	cub	cash
Kit	Kim	cab
cot	cup	kid

cut	cob	cap
cod	cat	cop
Kip	kin	cub

Kim had the cat on her lap.

Dad had a nap on the cot.

Did Jim cut his lip on this cup?

ck

lock	duck	back
pack	Nick	luck
sick	rock	puck

Rick	sock	tack
rack	Rick	tick
pick	lick	sack

Rick sat on the big rock.

Kim had bad luck.

The duck is back on the ship.

e

met	Meg	fed
let	leg	led
red	set	peck

Ben	bed	bet
pet	neck	shed
get	jet	beg

Meg fed her pet cat.

Did Ben sit on the deck?

Deb met her dad in his lab.

j, c, k, ck, e

1   Pat led the pup to his dish.

2   Ben had a bad cut on his leg.

3   Rob and Rick had to rush to get the bus.

4   Meg had a red hat but Rick did not.

5   Let the cat lick the dish.

6   Jim and Ben met in the shop.

7   The duck on the dock has a bad leg.

8   Kim did not jog with Mom.

9   Get Sid the red sock on the rug.

10   Jack and the dog got on the bus.

v, w, x, y, z

wag	wig	wish
vat	vet	Viv
zip	zag	zap

wet	yet	yes
fox	tax	box
wax	tux	Max

Did Jack wax his hot rod?

I wish Max had a dog.

Yes, the wig is on Viv.

ch, th

chop	rich	Chet
chip	chin	chap
chat	such	Chip

Beth	bath	thin
path	thick	thud
with	math	thug

Did Beth chop the log?

Chet had such fun with the pup.

Did Jim jog on the path?

qu, wh

quick	quack	quiz
quit	whip	when
whiz	whop	which

quit	when	quiz
whip	quick	whiz
quack	which	whop

When will Rick go to the vet with the pup?

Rick had a quick chat with Dad.

I wish that I had the quiz.

1 Is Jack in his tux?

2 The fox is in the pen with the hen.

3 Quick, run to get the wig!

4 Did that duck quack?

5 He was a whiz on that quiz.

6 The gal with the dog is Viv.

7 I wish to jog on that path.

8 Yes, Tom is a thin chap.

9 That pup had a hot bath.

10 The box of gum is with Dad.

mop	rib	sob
jog	rash	map
rock	cop	such
dot	lid	mud
Ted	fix	lap

web	not	lick
much	ten	quit
chip	tub	bed
moth	at	hip
lock	peg	shot

had	rich	bug
pen	bat	hit
pet	lash	bus
bun	pick	path
bib	red	jab
kid	nod	but
cup	mix	pot
Ben	kick	pat
tick	tab	Jim
tin	cob	rat

big	tip	cot
Rick	shut	dash
whip	mad	den
gum	math	neck
dip	mug	rush

sub	dish	wig
yes	fun	map
this	zip	sick
tug	pet	thin
cub	fit	hip

shut	rush	wish
quit	back	pup
fog	shop	sob
lot	hut	dash
jog	pack	sit

whip	let	gap
fish	sip	dug
rich	dig	cab
Sid	Rick	lot
vet	wax	chin

sock	shed	led
dug	mat	lit
pig	pup	nap
quit	kit	Gus
Jack	then	job

did	zap	rub
ship	tot	pad
fish	zag	rug
them	pal	fox
nut	gas	him

chug	vat	dab
pub	con	hub
sash	dim	pod
tax	dock	sag
lab	Sis	pin

pun	quip	hack
fib	shin	sag
mod	deck	chub
yen	quiz	chum
nick	sod	posh

yap	pug	thud
lack	sash	bob
hut	shag	tick
bud	hex	bog
hag	mob	hush

peck	hash	bid
sum	lush	rack
pod	lad	bin
dud	nog	rap
jack	cod	lag

pub	dim	vim
hem	wick	nun
kin	lug	dab
whiz	sack	sin
rid	fin	sag

nag	nab	yak
gal	rum	mesh
rig	shod	thug
rim	jut	shun
tux	chat	lax

gut	kin	mesh
chap	sop	shim
ped	hem	shin
cad	rut	fad
gag	keg	jot

mod	gum	bid
gap	tog	lox
gab	bin	lob
whim	wit	bop
whack	shun	jag

sut	vid	weg
kiz	zat	dep
pob	dem	vib
sot	lix	quib
yut	jeb	zeg

fub	gad	quop
med	dex	jid
ret	fap	piz
lig	wog	quat
jit	lub	hup

vin	gaz	min
dob	vob	wex
riz	tup	jux
dap	zib	foz
fif	quat	tex

bup	sep	jum
rop	ked	bish
lat	quap	chib
huz	feg	sith
quet	kiz	wup

tez	fep	lat
rem	gup	rab
dax	quop	choz
tem	poth	mip
yim	jup	bep

hosh	dith	wog
wib	yeb	fash
gom	vash	bix
jud	chep	dop
mish	chez	lod

1   Tim hid the cat in the shed.

2   The fish on that dish is hot.

3   Tim got the mop and the rag.

4   Tim and his pal, Tom, got the big job.

5   Tim had a nap.

6   Bob got a cut on his lip.

7   Beth had a wig and a hat.

8   Ted met Bev at the shop.

9   A big moth is in the pot.

10 Did Rick hop on that bus?

1   Jack did a jig on the rug.

2   Mom got the tot a bib.

3   Did Tom nab the fish with his rod?

4   Tim had a sip of pop.

5   Did the dog nip Pat?

6   Beth and Liz had to get the bus.

7   Ted got in the tub and had a bath.

8   Bob led the big dog to the dish.

9   Sal had a red dot on his chin.

10   The pen is not in the den.

1   The pig bit the hog in the hip.

2   The cat got the rat and bit him.

3   Bob had a mat on the big cot.

4   Did Chet wish that he had a pup?

5   Bob got in the tub for a bath.

6   The kid with Tom is not Rob.

7   Tim hit his chin and cut his lip.

8   It is a cub on the path!

9   Mom got fish and pop.

10   Tom got the gum on the rug.

1 Jim can not run on the thin path.

2 Tim got a nip from the pup.

3 Tom got a dish for his pet dog.

4 Ben let the dog on the bed.

5 Ted did not get the fish.

6 Max, pin a big rag to the mop.

7 Tim fed the cat six fish!

8 Sid sat in the hot tub for a bath.

9 The fox got the hen.

10 Peg did not get the pig in the pen.

1   Dad let Chet pack the bag.

2   Rick had a bad cut on his leg.

3   Shut the hen in the shed so that the dog does not get it.

4   Ed got the red fish with his net.

5   Did Ben get a nip on his neck from the pet?

6   Don dug a pit in the mud with Chad.

7   Did the dog wag and yap?

8   I wish to get that hat back for Tom.

9   Get the bug in the web.

10 Which jet did Ted get in?

1 Yes, Meg had to jog on that path.

2 Tom hit Jim in the rib.

3 Did Tom get the job at the sub shop?

4 Mom and Pat will gab and gab.

5 I will hush the mob.

6 Pat is a rich kid.

7 Dad did not get much cash for the job.

8 Jim is in the shed with Jack.

9 Pat will jog in the fog.

10 The rim of this pot is hot.

1 Tom got the map from the cab.

2 It is at the lab.

3 Bob and Jim will mop the rig.

4 Ben is such a nag at the shop that I wish he would quit the job!

5 Beth led Gus to sit and chat at the dock.

6 Did the vet dip the dog in the tick bath?

7 A yak dug in wet sod for a fig.

8 Tim will jab and hit the bag.

9 Did Kim rip the top of the rag?

10 Tom will jog on the path to the hut.

1   This job is big, but it is fun.

2   Mom did not nag Pat.

3   Chad had a nap on the cot.

4   The tot got a hug from his mom.

5   Tom got a jack and a lug nut for the job.

6   The thug hit Jim in the gut.

7   Rick will chop the log and lug it to the hut.

8   Meg and Bob sat and had a chat.

9   Beth had to get to the job at ten.

10 Chet got mad at his sis, Beth.

1 Don got mud on his hot rod.

2 Ed had bad jet lag.

3 Ted got a bid in for the ship.

4 Did Ed dash to the shop to get a bag of chips and dip?

5 Nick and Liz did yak and yak.

6 Yes, Ben is in a rut at his job.

7 Did Viv sob when she got the bad rap?

8 The vet had a shot for the dog.

9 Tom quit the job at the ship.

10 When did Beth get lax with the job?

1   That tax on gas is not bad.

2   Yes, Max did wish to get an A in math.

3   Did Jed lack vim for the job?

4   Bob got up to wax the hot rod.

5   Zax, the pup, is a lot of fun.

6   The Red Sox had to win!

7   Mr. Quin was at the dock at ten to get the ship.

8   Max got six fish with his rod.

9   The fox got the hen in the pen.

10   Did Ms. Lin get the bus at ten a.m.?

The Hat

Tim had a hat. The cat got the hat and Tim had a fit. The cat hid the hat. Then Tim got the hat and gave a pat to the cat.

Cod Fish

Beth got Ben a red net at the shop. Then Ben got a big fish in the net. It was a cod fish. Ben fed the fish to his pet cat, Jed. Jed did lap up the dish of cod fish.

Sid, Meg and Ben

Sid and Meg met Ben at the bus. Meg wanted to go to the shop, but Ben and Sid did not wish to go. Meg got them to go. At the shop, Meg let Sid get gum for Ben. Then Ben, Meg and Sid sat on a log in the sun.

The Pup

Ben had a wish. It was for a pup. Dad got a pup for Ben. Ben called the pup Mod. Mod did wag and yap.

Ben had to get the pup to the vet. The vet had a shot for Mod. Mod did nip the vet, yet the vet did not get mad. Then the pup did wag and yap again.

The Big Job

Kim and Bob got a big job. Kim and Bob had to mop the lab. At the lab, Kim got a rag. Bob got a mop and a hot pot. The lab was then tip-top.

Cut Lip

Mom got the tot, Jim, a bib. Jim bit the fig and bit his lip. He had a sip of pop. His lip was OK. Then, Jim got on the mat with his pal, the cat.

Beth and the Pup

On the job, at the shop, Beth had a pal. It was a pup. The pup was a lost dog. It did wag and yap. Beth led the pup to a dish. The pup then sat with Beth. Beth called the pup "Zip".

Jim and Kim

Kim had a lot of fun at the shop. She got a top for Jim but it did not fit him. Jim had to go back to the shop with the top. When he was at the shop, he got a top that fit, then he got a pin for Kim.

The Fox

A fox got in the hen pen. Mr. Quin and Viv had to get the fox. They hid in the shed. Mr. Quin had a bad leg. At six, the fox got on top of the pen. When Viv got mad, the fox ran.

The Jog

Jim got up to jog on the path. It was not hot so Jim did a lap. A big log was on the path. Jim fell in a rut on the path and hit his chin on the log. The run was not much fun.

The Bash

Ted is mad at Liz and Liz is mad at Ted. At the bash, Liz did gab and gab to Don. Then Ted did nab Don and bop him in the rib. Liz had a fit. It was a big mix up. Liz and Don were just pals, but Ted did not want Liz to be with him at the bash.

Tim at the Sub Shop

Tim sat in the sub shop. A mom and a tot came in the shop. The mom got gum for the tot. Then a kid came in the shop. The kid got a can of pop and a sub. Then a gal came in the shop. The gal did not get gum or pop. The gal came to see Tim. The gal was Liz. Liz did yak and yak.

The Shop is Hit

Tim sat at the shop. A man with a bag came in. The man came up to Tim. Tim did not run. Tim had to put cash in the bag. Then the bad man ran. Tim was sad, but he had to get a cop and let him in the shop.

Tim and the Cop

The cop came in the shop. Tim told him about the bad man with the bag. The man was not fat and he was not thin. He had a red rash on his chin. He had a cap with a big dot on it. The cop had to jot this on his pad. Then the cop had to get the man and the cash.

hog	led	shell
cuff	shut	fuss
pit	miss	sad
will	moth	kiss
rap	dig	mad

lid	wish	pill
off	bit	fill
puff	toss	met
doll	sat	miss
hid	hill	rag

fell	gush	Chet
chill	rip	Russ
yell	Meg	Ken
Bess	huff	pop
well	kiss	mess

rot	Nell	chug
wall	chop	mass
nip	log	bell
bath	pill	will
call	huff	ball

dull	chess	tall
moss	keg	dill
mill	buff	bill
miss	shag	hall
gag	hiss	fib

gab	miff	fall
gap	ball	sill
lob	muff	lass
call	lull	joss
till	wall	mall

thill	poff	fass
raff	tuss	yill
poss	sull	siff
vell	jull	goss
hoff	liss	vull

hess	tull	daff
kell	niff	wess
zuff	rass	lill
rull	sess	zuff
faff	zall	biss

1 I will huff and puff up the big hill.

2 Bill is well, but he has been sick.

3 Did Chet get the red shell?

4 Bess had a big kiss for her dad.

5 This hall is a mess!

6 Mom did not miss the mud at all.

7 Ken fell on the path.

8 Toss the ball to Kim.

9 Will Jill and Russ go to the mall?

10 Can you call the pup for his bath?

1 Beth sat in the den with Bill.

2 Tim will fill the dish with fish.

3 Bill had to mop up the mess.

4 The bug fell in the web.

5 Did Dad yell at Tom?

6 Bev got a chill in the tub.

7 Jack had to sell his pig and his hog.

8 Ed will kill the big bug in the den.

9 Bess got Tom to go to the mall.

10 Dad had the red ball for Jen.

1 Did Jill hiss at the bad dog?

2 Dad will fill the cup with pop.

3 Ben had fun with the lass.

4 Ted will not jog in this fog.

5 Bob had a big kiss from Meg.

6 Will Liz get that dull job?

7 I bet Nell will pass in math.

8 The lass will get the bill at the pub.

9 Did Rick pass the hot rod at the top
of the hill?

10 Jill and Ted will kiss and tell.

1   The wig had fuzz and moss on top.

2   The lass hid on the hill.

3   Did Jim miss Liz when she got a new job?

4   Beth will fill the pot on the sill with sod.

5   The boss got a bell for the shop.

6   Jeff did not yell at the tot when he got gum on the rug.

7   Sal got Liz a chess set at the West Mall.

8   I bet that job was dull.

9   The call was from Kim's dad.

10 His pal, Sid, fell in the hall.

A Cut Lip

Bill was with his dad when he fell off the log. He bit his lip when his chin hit the log. The cut was not bad, but Bill was sad. His dad had a kit with him. It had a pad to rub on the cut.

The Big Hit

Russ had to get his sis, Jill, up from a nap. Russ and Jill had to get the bus to go to see the Red Sox. Russ and Jill sat in the sun. Russ got a hot dog. Then the bat hit the ball with a thud. The mob did yell. Yes! It was a big hit over the wall. The Red Sox did win.

Ben and Ted

Ben and Ted had fun. They got gas in the hot rod and set off. At the top of the hill, Ben did pass a cab. Then Ben did a dash to the mall. At the mall, Ben and Ted met Pat and Bess. They sat and had a chat. It was fun.

Zip

Beth went home. Zip, the pup, went with Beth. Beth gave Jeff a kiss. Then Zip sat on Beth's lap. Jeff did not want a pet, but Zip was such a sad pup that Jeff said OK. Beth then had to fill the tub so Zip could get a bath.

Beth and Liz Shop

Beth and Liz got the bus. They had to shop at the mall. Beth had to get a hat and Liz had to get a chess set for her dad. They had pops and a fish dish at the pub. Beth and Liz had to huff and puff to get the bus. They did not wish to miss it.

ham	pass	leg
Sam	can	yell
Beth	than	shell
fuss	Ned	cash
pan	sell	Seth

did	Jan	am
leg	than	tell
jam	Dan	tap
had	met	Don
tan	mix	Pam

fog	can	sun
bet	ham	run
Chad	fan	man
sap	sham	kill
ped	jut	rob

ban	fen	rod
jot	yum	gull
bam	chum	dam
shun	vat	bash
man	ram	yam

zam	lan	tiv
zat	vam	laz
han	bap	hud
kem	yex	yan
roff	quam	fam

heg	gop	zan
kep	lib	bam
cax	san	jun
quan	yab	pesh
tham	shan	cham

1   Jill can nap on the bed.

2   Dan sat in the pig pen!

3   The dog ran a path to get the cat.

4   Pat hid the jam in the shed.

5   Did Beth get the fan for the hot den?

6   Sam will get in the tub for a hot bath.

7   The ram on the hill is big.

8   Ben had a red and tan hat.

9   Pam and Bob had fun at the mill with dad.

10   Sam has a bad rash on his leg.

1 Did Pam get that wig at the shop?

2 Dad will dash to get the ham.

3 The moth fell in the yam.

4 I am sad about the Red Sox loss.

5 Can Liz and Rich do the job?

6 Ed and Tom will jam in the shed.

7 Dan had to rush the pup to a vet.

8 The man got a cash tip for the job.

9 Mash that yam in the pan.

10 Seth had ham with his egg.

Pam and Jam

Pam had to get jam for her dad. She ran to the shop. It did not have jam. She ran to see Liz. Liz did not have jam. Then she got a bus to the Big D shop. The Big D had jam! Pam got the jam for her dad. Dad had the jam and a big kiss for Pam.

The Fan

It was such a hot day! Dan sat in the den. The den was hot. Dan did not sit – he got up. It was too hot. Dan had to get the fan.

Sam was in bed for a nap and he had the fan. Dan got the fan. Then Sam got hot and got up from his nap. Dan was in the den with his fan. Sam was then mad at Dan.

dogs	pens	pups
shops	locks	webs
nets	pegs	hams
wins	chins	backs
mats	mills	chills

maps	tops	bugs
sips	wets	bills
rubs	necks	bells
lugs	shuts	rugs
shells	fans	tins

kicks	huffs	sheds
wins	pins	runs
fills	nuts	packs
jugs	sits	bugs
pats	zags	naps

tubs	buds	sets
fibs	dads	socks
pills	chips	ships
dabs	kids	paths
pits	cans	quits

subs	kits	whips
puns	mobs	docks
yams	bins	nags
pecks	lads	chums
robs	yells	racks
thugs	sums	yens
decks	peds	rigs
quills	rots	lacks
tics	dubs	jabs
hags	pecks	huts

zups	wegs	yips
baps	mips	cheds
tods	duts	sans
lems	rills	jops
kigs	gans	vams

shids	thons	wubs
zugs	hets	fams
foms	whibs	chots
biffs	daths	zums
shens	mabs	thubs

nugs	duts	mons
quebs	zans	luns
dods	jegs	sibs
qualls	rabs	fums
chims	heffs	shobs

whabs	puds	chigs
tibs	queds	gogs
yats	juffs	thims
shens	valls	yans
futs	fams	thigs

1 Dad sits in the den and pets Whim, his dog.

2 The kids nap on the cot.

3 Tim got the mops and rags in the shed.

4 The rugs had lots of mud on them.

5 Mr. Quin yells at the kids.

6 Seth runs to the dock with his six big fish.

7 Ben sells dolls in his shop.

8 The shells are red when they get wet.

9 Chet lugs the jug up the hill.

10 Pam hugs the pup when it is sad.

1 Don's dog, Sam, has ticks.

2 The kids get chips at the shop.

3 Mom fills the jugs in the shed.

4 Bob naps in the den on the rug.

5 Jim has bags of shells for the tots.

6 Chet gabs to Jill as she sips pop.

7 The kids had the ball in the bin.

8 Fill the jug with the nuts.

9 The dog runs with Tim.

10 Did you get the bells for the shop?

1   Mom nods to Jim to get Sis.

2   Tom runs to the bus in such a rush.

3   Fill the cups with pop for the kids.

4   Al will mop the decks and the hall.

5   The decks of the ship get lots of sun.

6   I miss my chums at the shop.

7   The hub caps are in the van.

8   Dan shops at the mall with Will.

9   Beth lugs the mops and rags.

10 The maps are not in the cab.

1   Yes, Viv is nuts about Bill!

2   Ed bops at the bash and has fun.

3   The thug got hub caps, but then the cops got him.

4   Sid quits a job if it is not fun.

5   Ben jabs the bag and then jogs.

6   The boss cons Beth to do the job.

7   Did the cops get the kids in the hot rod?

8   Bill nags Tom to fix the hub caps on his rig.

9   Meg gets the chills when she is in the pit.

10 The fans yell for Nick at bat.

Hot Dogs and Pops

Sam sells a lot of hot dogs and pops on hot days. When it is hot, kids get lots. Then Sam gets lots of cash. When it is not hot, Sam has a bad day. So, Sam will wish for the sun.

Max

Max quits jobs on a whim. If he gets mad at the boss, he quits. If he is sad, he quits. If he has the wish to get his chums and have fun, he quits. This is bad for Max. He will not get the cash for his bills. Max will not get rich!

Posttest Step 1

A

pan	quit	fix
bud	ham	shell
chips	locks	path
miss	nets	huff
rush	fall	maps

B

chess	vat	yams
hex	dull	decks
quip	miff	rips
whims	sham	van
pits	yen	walls

Posttest Step 1

Nonsense Words

fams	shup	rez
zops	gud	veb
hin	wheps	jith
luns	quess	rills
hux	nans	wubs

1 Words with a suffix: Underline the basewords and circle the suffix.

2 Circle the "chicken" letter.

3 Underline or highlight digraphs.

4 Box "welded" sounds.

5 Put a star (★) above "bonus" letters.

NOTES

NOTES

NOTES